The Essential Oils Weight Loss Solution

5 Minute Aromatherapy Recipes for Burning Fat, Shedding Pounds, and Feeling Great!

Fiona Summers

Just to say thank you for purchasing this book, I'd like to give you a gift. It's completely free and is invaluable for anyone using essential oils.

You won't want to miss it!

To download, click visit:

fionasummers.com

DISCLAIMER

All rights reserved. No part of this publication or the information in it may be quoted from or reproduced in any form by means such as printing, scanning, photocopying or otherwise without prior written permission of the copyright holder.

Terms of Use: This book has been written by a professionally qualified and practicing aromatherapist. Although the author and publisher have made every effort to ensure that the information in this book is accurate and complete, they do not warrant the accuracy of the information, text and graphics contained within the book due to the rapidly changing nature of science, research, known and unknown facts and internet.

The Author and the publisher do not hold any responsibility for errors, omissions or contrary interpretation of the subject matter herein. This book is presented solely for motivational and informational purposes only.

For further details please see the detailed safety information on page 61 and a full disclaimer on page 71 before using this book.

Summary

This book takes an in-depth look into why your body has become fat and what you can do to change it. It uses methods used by trained aromatherapists but is written as a simple to follow manual to be used by anyone, even complete aromatherapy beginners.

It begins by looking at how toxins lodge in your fat cells, binding them to your body. Whilst the toxins remain, it is impossible for that fat to be burned away.

It then relates oils which clear these toxins and allow the physical body to start burning calories more effectively. It also explores how your brain is conspiring against you, making it difficult for you to shed pounds. It lists essential oils and other therapies to cleanse both mind and body...and make them work like the much slimmer you.

Discover how to choose your essential oils wisely. Get the best quality available for the least amount of money.

Lastly are some sample recipes to help you begin your treatment plan.

Nothing could be easier. And, of course, it's 100% safe.

In fact...using essential oils to lose weight is a piece of cake when you have read this book.

Contents

1. **An Age Old Secret Revealed At Last**.......................8
2. **The Holistic Approach**..............................13
3. **The Physiology of Weight Loss**......................16
   - Thyroid 17
   - Adrenal Glands 18
   - Pituitary 19
   - Hypothalamus 20
   - Liver 22
   - Gall Bladder 24
   - Pancreas 24
   - Kidney 25
   - Circulation 26
   - Lymphatic System 27
   - Muscles 28
4. **Obesity and the Emotions**...........................29
   - Issues in the Tissues..30
   - Night Eating Syndrome 31
   - Internalising Negative Social Stigma 31
   - Affirmations For Weight Loss 32
   - Oils for the Emotions 36
   - Other emotional oils for your list 36
   - Oils to fight off lethargy 38
5. **Natural Therapies for Weight Loss**..................39
   - How to use essential oils 42
   - Inhalation 42

Through the skin 43

Discover Carrier oils 44

In The Bath 44

Creams and Lotions 45

Burners 45

Dilution and Blending 46

Clays 46

Green Clay 47

Red clay 47

Sea Weed 47

Sea Salt Therapy 48

Lymphatic Drainage 49

Acupressure points 51

Phytotherapy and Herbal Suggestions 53

Anti Cellulite Diet 53

6. Housekeeping 55

Buying essential oils 56

Storing Essential Oils 59

Safety Advice 61

7. Recipes 62

Willpower Evaporator Oil 63

Resilience Lotion 63

Environmental Cleansing Massage Oil 63

Fat Burning Lotion 64

Bye Bye Hunger Pangs Lotion (For Daytime Use) 64

Bye Bye Hunger Pangs Lotion (For Evening Use) 65

Stress Cleanse 65

Inch Loss Wrap 66
   Skin Tightening Gel 66
Conclusion **68**
Bibliography **69**
Disclaimer **71**

1. An Age Old Secret Revealed At Last

In 1982, a book called The Practice of Aromatherapy was published by Dr Jean Valnet. Considered to be the father of aromatherapy, he wrote copious notes about plants and their healing abilities. Considered to be one of the most important works in holistic medicine, it is still recommended on aromatherapy reading lists.

He writes of an extraordinary feat of healing, involving a dreadfully obese teenager and how he was able to overcome the child's problems using essential oils. Sadly he omitted to explain which oils were used! This book fills in the gaps of which plant essences are able to bring about these effects.

It explains how essential oils and plant extracts can be used to kick start the body into shedding pounds quicker and more effectively. It replaces some elements of Valnet's regime with more accessible and palatable alternatives and brings together the very best in healing practices to ensure you lose the largest number of pounds possible for your time at the gym.

Let's be honest, if you are going to have lettuce for lunch and skip that chocolate éclair dessert, you want to know it's going to be worth it don't you?!

First, I'll let Dr Valnet tell you about his remarkable feat.

Case No. 3 – Obesity in an adolescent

B, a youth aged 16, weighed 85kg about 13 ½ stone for a height of 1m 62 (5ft 4ins). The basal metabolic rate had fallen to -6%. Various treatments had been tried without effect, and the boy like his family was desperate.

In July 1961 he was treated with phyto and aromatherapy, thyroid treatments and sea water. Naturally, bread, cakes, pastries and delicatessen foods were forbidden.

In February 1961 he was given packed cell therapy. Three months later, young B had lost 17kg (more than 21/2 stone) in weight.

These results were confirmed in September 1970, no further treatment having been necessary-indeed the diet had been long since abandoned. At the age of 25 the patient was in perfect health and possessed of Herculean strength, his height was 1m 73 cm (5ft 8ins) and his weight 74kg (roughly 11½ stone)

Dr Jean Valnet: The Practice of Aromatherapy

Taking a guess, there might be several terms people will be unfamiliar with.

Phytotherapy is quite an antiquated term which has suddenly re-found popularity. It covers all manner of plant medicines from herbalism to aromatherapy, flower essences and the use of sea weeds, clays and tissue salts. This book will show you how to manipulate the bodily hormones using all manner of plant extracts.

This book is written with a strong bias towards aromatherapy for several reasons. The first is, for a beginner, it is a very simple and quite inexpensive healing mechanism to use. Once the oils are absorbed through the skin into the blood stream they get to work healing. Dosage is very straightforward and is difficult to get wrong.

In some ways plant medicine is safer than the doctor's traditional pills and lotions because there are no side effects of the treatments. Conversely though, every plant medicine has many main effects (for example lavender is relaxing, as well as soothing to the skin. Cardamom is sedative, but it is also laxative so you could start visiting the toilet more often without knowing why) so it is important not to trigger too many hormones all at once. Focusing on aromatherapy helps us to avoid doing this.

By far the biggest advantage though is essential oils are skin absorbed. There is no need to take any oral treatments, which is a much safer option without the supervision of a qualified therapist.

I have however covered some very basic supplementary therapies which will help you to boost the essential oils capacity to help you lose weight in a safe and measured way.

Packed cell therapy is a way to replace blood supply and replenish it with new fresh supplies. Nowadays this is only used for very severe blood emergencies; it usually takes the form of transfusion. This book, rather than hooking you up to a bag of O Neg explains how to naturally encourage your circulation to work more effectively in order to process fats faster.

Sea water therapy is a great idea for people who live on the coast, but for the rest of us it is pretty difficult. Instead we explain how you can use both salt and sea weed in different ways to bring about the same effects. Better than that we find ways where you need not ingest the salt if you don't fancy it!

Unlike traditional medicine though, holistic medicine does not only treat the symptom of the fat tummy and ever widening hips, it seeks to isolate and treat the reasons your problems may have occurred in the first place. The next chapter explains how this works better than anything you will find in the pharmacy.

2. The Holistic Approach

Scientists have discovered that environmental toxins absorbed from the air, water, soil, food and even the drugs we take go into our bodies and then get stuck there. They are stored in two main places, in your liver and in fat storage deposits around our body. Main holistic practitioners agree the reason the terrifying fact these toxins are playing such a massive part in obesity and diabetes is not headline news, is because the doctors have not yet created a drug to fight it.

Holistic medicine looks at the entire person rather than the symptoms they exhibit. Many factors have lead to that spare tyre you are sporting. Emotions which may be causing you to over eat, glands not firing as they should of course these wicked toxins no-one's talking about.

50 years ago the treatments in this book would have been discounted as quack medicine. 200 years ago, rather than essential oils, it is likely they would be the fresh herbs used. Now, however, aromatherapy and plant medicines (phytotherapy) are accepted as almost main stream. So how did things come full circle?

Well healing didn't change, attitudes did. The world saw how a synthetic drug like Penicillin could save lives and it jumped on the traditional medicine band wagon. Unknown to many people, many of our hospital drugs started their lives as plant. Digitalis originally came from fox gloves, Valium from the valiant plants and morphine came from poppies.

Cleverly, scientists identified the active constituents and synthesized that one part of the plant.

Now whilst on one hand this genius move was able to save not only many lives but also time and money, it came with its own problems. When an entire plant is used it is a complete medicine with its own stabilizing effects; it has many main effects. Synthesizing plant extracts has a side effect, and that is side effects - Addiction being one of the main ones.

So, these are the secrets the drug companies don't want you to know. Not only can you get slim for a fraction of the time and effort, but cost doesn't even come into it. Plant medicine is cheap, it is healthy and it's not licensed to make drug company fat cats!

3. THE PHYSIOLOGY OF WEIGHT LOSS

Thyroid

You may often hear people claim their weight gain is due to an underactive thyroid gland. This could be true. Then again it may not be - it could also be down to a few too many donuts, and a sedentary lifestyle. Often it is difficult to tell.

Your doctor is able to perform tests to confirm suspicions but sadly the levels of dysfunction have to be extreme to register on his scale. Even small levels of dysfunction can cause weight gain and other symptoms too.

Given this then, let's use this as your starting point.

What is the thyroid?

This is found at the base of the neck and is primarily its job is metabolism. It is part of a complex set of <u>glands</u> called the endocrine system, whose job it is to control the hormone levels in your body. Imagine your endocrine system a bit like a row of dominos, if one drops out of kilter it affects the next, then the next and the next. Look for other glands in the list which will also be participating in your endocrine's function.

If you have an underactive thyroid you will be prone to pile on the weight very quickly but also be very susceptible to the cold. Potentially you may be moaning about temperature changes than others around you.

Over activity of this gland can make people very over excitable and anxious. Your heartbeat and breathing may also be extremely rapid. Serious over secretion causes a build up in the neck and creates an enlarged throat in a condition called goitre. This is rarely seen nowadays, but it used to be called Derbyshire Neck because it was endemic in that area of England as well as in the Alps. Later it was discovered there was a lack of iodine in the water in these areas which had caused the thyroid to cease to regulate effectively.

Essential Oils which affect the Thyroid: Myrrh balances the production of thyroxin, Clove, Lemongrass and Peppermint are also indicated. Black Spruce is effective in the treatment of hyperthyroidism

These oils are best applied over the thymus which sits just underneath your sternum in the middle of your rib cage.

Adrenal Glands

These are situated on top of your kidneys. They produce a number of different hormones involved in many different body processed.

The adrenals secrete adrenaline which is produced as part of our Fight or Flight Syndrome." It quickens the breathing and heart rate. When an athlete prepares for a race, these nervous reactions are vital for gorging the muscles with enough blood to make them as powerful as they can be. Originally this was useful for outrunning a sabre-toothed tiger but now if we learn to use it effectively it is a powerful mechanism for ensuring we are on top of our game. Problems occur of course when the body does not know how to shut off and bring down the levels back again.

Imagine having a crash, or even someone puts the phone down on you, the urge to scream and shout does not leave you. There is no "closure" to use a very 90s word. It has been suggested that the bloke who gets out of his car and smashes the man who reversed into him actually has a more healthy response than the more careful soul who takes insurance details. He found an outlet for the energy surge and as such the levels can drop.

This is a classic example of how the endocrine glands domino out of control. As you read on, you will see how stress leads to what possibly is your worst enemy…comfort eating.

Essential Oils which affect the adrenals:

Mandarin, Camomile Maroc,

PITUITARY
It had previously thought this gland was the manager of the endocrine system but recent research has shown it does have a boss. It is influenced by the workings of the hypothalamus which we will investigate more in the next section. For the purposes of simplicity I want you to consider the pituitary to be the foreman this complex factory.

The majority of the hormones which are secreted by the pituitary are to do with fertility and sexuality so on the surface it would seem the pituitary plays no part. What is important to note here is any long term stress drains the adrenals which then drags energy from your pituitary which then in turn is like an energetic parasite to your hypothalamus.

Before we move on I will also add the pituitary is essential to the health of the ovaries and testes. Clearly if your libido has dropped, are suffering bouts of impotence, the pituitary needs further assessment. In terms of obesity too though, Poly Cystic Ovarian Syndrome (PCOS) directly relates to the pituitary. I will address this more in the section about the ovaries.

The best tonic for the pituitary is nutmeg oil (also sprinkle the ground spice on your food).

HYPOTHALAMUS
This small structure situated inside of the brain exerts its main influence over the nervous system and is generally believed to be involved with appetite. It controls hunger, thirst, sexual response and also temperature. It is linked with the brain but also with the pituitary too. It serves as an interface between the mind, the central nervous system, the autonomic nervous system and the hormone producing glands.

The hypothalamus is now known to be the missing piece of the jigsaw explaining how the way we are feeling can affect our health. As the emotions change, messages pass through the hypothalamus which then translate through to the glands and then in turn, affect the organs.

Are you able to see how step by step stress can be causing your weight gain?

Essential oils which affect the Hypothalmus are:

For temperature and appetite issues: peppermint or ginger

To align the mind body spirit- Frankincense

One of the main organs affected not only by stress, but poor diet and lack of exercise too, is the liver.

LIVER

The liver is the foreman of the body. It has many functions which are:

- The production of bile. This helps carry away waste and break down fats in the small intestine during digestion

- The production of certain proteins for blood plasma

- It is involved in the production of cholesterol and special proteins which help carry fats through the body

- It converts excess glucose into glycogen for storage (This glycogen can later be converted back to glucose for energy.)

- It regulates blood levels of amino acids. These form the building blocks of proteins

- It processes haemoglobin for use of its iron content (The liver stores iron.)

- It converts poisonous ammonia to urea (Urea is one of the end products of protein metabolism which is excreted in urine.)

- It clears the blood of drugs and other poisonous substances

- It regulates blood clotting

- It builds resistance to infection by producing immune factors and removing bacteria from the blood stream

The liver relies very heavily on the adrenals to know how to perform. When the adrenals become depleted of energy the liver quickly follows suit. There are other protagonists too which will affect your liver performance.

- Food: The food we eat nowadays is in the main, not as good as it used to be. Because of intensive farming with fertilisers and petrochemicals, most of our crops (and indeed in some parts of the world the air we breathe) are laden with heavy metals. The human body has never been able to assimilate itself to be able to the deal with these "new" synthetic toxins and they lodge themselves within the liver.

- Alcohol…no need to labor that point.

- Vitamin B deficiency: The body needs Vitamin B to fuel the liver. If the liver has to work extra hard to compensate for the adrenals being so exhausted it will burn even more of it. Add to that the substandard nutrient levels in our processed food and the body simply cannot make enough to keep up. I can recommend a daily supplement of 100mg daily.

Astounding how many things it does, isn't it? Can you see how the liver has his thumb in every ones pie? If your liver becomes dysfunctional it will affect a whole range of different organs but in particular your gall bladder, your kidneys and also your circulatory system.

ESSENTIAL OILS FOR THE LIVER
Eucalyptus, camomile maroc, peppermint, rosemary

OILS FOR CHOLESTEROL
Rosemary oil is proven to reduce cholesterol and also is thought to curb hunger too. This oil however causes seizures in sufferers of epilepsy.

GALL BLADDER
The gall bladder is predominately a storage organ for bile. For those who do not know bile breaks down fats and also helps the body to rid itself of toxins. As the bile sits in the gall bladder it becomes more and more concentrated in order that it be able to attack fats more effectively.

Essential oils which affect the gall bladder are: Fennel, Calendula, Ginger

PANCREAS
Many of you will recognise the correlation between the onset of Type 2 Diabetes and obesity, but how does this happen?

The job of the pancreas is to process enzymes which break down fats in the form of juices. A healthy pancreas is able to produce juices at the right times to be able to manage the foods we eat. Inside of the pancreas these is a gland called the Islet of Langerhans which manufactures insulin in response to a rise in blood sugar.

Overeating stresses the internal parts of the cells called the Endoplasmic rectilium, which then send out distress signals to dampen down the insulin receptors on the cell. This is what causes someone to become Insulin Resistant. It also explains why diabetes can be reversed using diet....all we are actually looking for is the cell to stop sending out distress signals.

A word of warning here for diabetic patients: essential oils affect the way the body processes blood sugar. Keep a close eye on your blood sugar levels; they may start to work differently to before you started using aromatherapy

Essential oils which affect the Islets of Langerhans are Helichrysm and Spearmint.

Kidney

The kidneys are the main control of the urinary system.

They are bean shaped and lie against the posterior wall about the height of the waist. The right kidney hangs lower than the left.

Their job is to filter out salt, water, urea and glucose from the blood. Considering how diverse our diet is you can imagine how complex a job this is. The average composition of urine is about 96% water and then 2% urea and 2% salts.

Urea can also be measured in blood plasma and in that form it makes up about 0.4% urea. This shows us that the concentration has increased by about 50 times by the time it has been processed by the kidneys. As blood circulates through the kidneys large quantities are filtered into The Capsules of Bowman. From here they are transported into tubules where all of the glucose and most of the water and salts are returned to the blood. Although the kidneys process around 150-180 litres of fluid in a day, only about 1.5 litres leave the body as urine.

Essential oils which affect the kidneys are: Black pepper, camomile maroc, cypress, fennel(sweet), Frankincense, Geranium, Ginger, jasmine, juniper, lavender, lemon, mandarin, marjoram, nutmeg, patchouli, rose, rosemary, spikenard, tea tree and ylang ylang.

CIRCULATION

This is almost back to front because predominately obesity will cause poor circulation. As you lose weigh though, encouraging the circulation will not only allow your body to detoxify faster but also help the excess skin to tighten too.

Essential oils which will help improve circulation are: Black Pepper, geranium and cypress.

Cardamom also improves the condition of the blood to help the nutrients of any vitamin supplements to absorb better.

Lymphatic System

It stands a chance that the women among you may be more familiar with the effects of lymphatic dysfunction than the gentlemen. Our old enemy cellulite is directly related to this, in other ways however its functions are not clearly evident.

It has three main functions. These are:

- To drain the fluid from the cells
- To distribute the fats and fat soluble nutrients
- To fight infection.

Already you should be able to see why this system will be important in your regime. In many ways it is similar to the circulatory system in that it moves fluid around your body; in circulation the fluid is blood, here it is colorless liquid called lymph. How the two systems differ is circulation is powered by a pump, the heart, whereas the lymphatic system relies on muscle tone and compression.

If you find the base of your collar bone, you can locate the subclavian vein which is one of two places lymphatic system empties. It runs down the side of the neck and along the bone. The head, neck, right arm and right side of the chest all drain into the right subclavian. The rest of the body drains into the left.

When the muscles themselves get to work, they produce waste, which in turn the lymphatic system removes from the body too.

Later in the book I will explain how we can emulate the effects of the muscles and encourage the lymphatic system to work more efficiently using a special massage technique. For now, it serves to say...another reason to get off the sofa and get working out. If nothing else you will know you are improving your immune system.

Oils for the lymphatic system are: Sandalwood, fennel, helichrysm, myrtle, lemongrass, tangerine and orange

MUSCLES

Your sedentary lifestyle may mean you have lost some muscle tone; there are problems with this apart from the fact you no longer look like Mr(s) Universe. The lymphatic system relies on muscular tone to work effectively.

Implementing the following oils into your treatment plan will really help to improve muscle tone: Ginger, Grapefruit, Sweet Marjoram, Pine, Rosemary

4. OBESITY AND THE EMOTIONS

Issues in the Tissues

We have seen how emotions can affect the internal workings of the body, but of course feelings play pretty horrid tricks on the mind too. Psychologists all agree weight problems are all intrinsically linked with feelings with low self esteem and self value. What one needs to ask, is which came first, the chicken or the egg?

In fact, statistics show the correlation is higher in women than men, with a massive 37% of obesity cases linked with depression. Certainly depression and anxiety are high protagonists and people who are overweight are much more likely to be associated with feelings of suicide.

This is an area for someone far more gifted than I so I shall not be arrogant enough to take on the role of a counsellor or psychologist here. What can be useful here though, is to write a food diary of everything you eat and when, along with the activities and feelings which you are experiencing at the time. Identifying triggers which can catapult you into raiding the fridge are extremely useful weapons in the fight against weight loss.

Advice from the American Psychological Association suggests tacking the emotions behind the eating can prove more effective than a diet alone.

Night Eating Syndrome

I was shocked when I read about this actual syndrome (abbreviated to NES) which affects around 1% of the population. Anyone who regularly consumes more than 35% of their daily calories after they have already had their evening meals, in 1955 this syndrome was identified as a problem with the sufferer's internal body clock.

Oils thought to stabilize the circadian rhythms are: Lavender, rose, rosemary and grapefruit.

Internalising Negative Social Stigma

By now you will be starting to have an understanding of how emotions may be affecting your health. Reacting to social stigma can be one of the most difficult aspects of weight gain you can face. For some reason these days, there are people who feel it is acceptable to comment on your size and perceived lack of will power. They say things loud and proud as if somehow your being larger than them makes them better and actually....makes you deaf!

Thinking back to adrenals and the example of someone slamming the phone down...let's change that to someone making snide comments about how long you are taking in front of them in the supermarket queue.

Most people want to run and hide when they are subject to such bullying, or even turn and punch them in the face....but you don't do you?

So again we are sending negative emotions straight to the adrenals, and we are adding these spiteful words to our own internal library of reasons why we don't deserve to look good and shine.

Just how many ways do we need to detox our minds and bodies? Welcome to the world of holistic healing....it goes on and on.

Let's think about how we detox and nourish our minds.

Affirmations For Weight Loss

Research shows that each day we have around 50,000 thoughts. Scarily for most of us, a massive 80% of those are negative.

Read that again.

Terrifying, isn't it?

Now above all things, your self esteem and belief is what is going to make you feel better about yourself, your body, your worthiness to love yourself and be loved. Feeling strong will get that weight off.

There are many affirmations floating around in cyber space and actually you could make up your own. These, however are flagrantly stolen from the website of a lady called Louise Hay, authoress of the book You Can Change Your Life. She is the original and the best! You will find loads more help from her site: http://www.healyourlifetraining.com/affirmations/weight-loss-affirmations

Spending a few moments a day repeating a couple of these 8-10 times helps your mind to start to believe these things are true. I promise you...every slender celebrity strutting her stuff on the red carpet feels just as unsettled about her body as you do now, but she understand the her own self worth. This is where you start to learn the same.

Every day my relationship with food becomes healthier.

I am learning and using the mental, emotional, and spiritual skills for success.

I am willing to change!

I love my body.

I appreciate my body.

It's exciting to discover my unique food and exercise system for weight loss.

I am delighted to be the ideal weight for me.

It's easy for me to follow a healthy food plan.

I choose to embrace thoughts of confidence in my ability to make positive changes in my life.

It feels good to move my body. Exercise is fun!

I use deep breathing to help me relax and handle stress.

I am a good person.

I deserve to be at my ideal weight.

I am a lovable person.

I deserve love.

It is safe for me to lose weight.

I am a strong presence in the world at my lower weight.

I accept and enjoy my sexuality.

It's OK to feel sensuous.

My metabolism is excellent.

You may also find hypnosis to be a great help. Not only will a good hypnotist help you strengthen your resolve to lose weight but also work on the unconscious triggers in the brain which are causing the hormone imbalances we have talked about.

OILS FOR THE EMOTIONS

ANGER
Rose, camomile, lavender, geranium, melissa

ANXIETY
Lavender, camomile, marjoram, geranium

DEPRESSION
Melissa, bergamot, ginger, rose

FEAR
Angelica (of dying), marjoram, camomile

FRUSTRATION
Thyme, geranium, bergamot

STRESS
To soothe: Lavender, camomile, geranium, rose

OTHER EMOTIONAL OILS FOR YOUR LIST
In her wonderful book Aromantics, Valerie Ann Worwood talks quite extensively about her experiences treating patients with problems overeating. She talks of BERGAMOT, which often

would be used to stimulate appetite (remember many main effects of an oil?) but how conversely the oil seemed to balance the appetite by dealing with the underlying emotions which had initially caused the issue.

ROSE is the very best investment you can make in rebuilding happiness in your life.

For those of you who are dodging the mirror, weight possibly is not your only issue. Use FRANKINCENSE to boost confidence, geranium to sooth frantic panic and Lemon Balm to put that smile back on your face. I promise you confidence is far sexier than any tiny frock.

In her book *The Garden of Eden, Jill Bruce* gives lots of ideas of oils which can make that subtle but powerful difference to your healing.

BENZOIN – Helps to unlock mental fetters which may be stopping you from achieving your goal.

CITRONELLA – Lifts the blues and sweetens the mood.

FENNEL (SWEET) – Gives patience

HELICHRYSM – Makes willpower more steadfast

LAVENDER (BULGARIAN) – Helps you get past the boredom of the diet.

MANDARIN – Steely resolve

MYRRH – Strengthening qualities, a little like the effects of prayer.

ORANGE – Helps you to see what you are truly capable of.

ROSE MAROC – Helps you be steadfast even when people knock your confidence.

ROSEWOOD – Useful if there are problems from peer pressure, especially for teenagers.

TAGETES – Gives stillness. Helps you to look inside of yourself to find strength.

OILS TO FIGHT OFF LETHARGY

The truth is no matter how much you try to kid yourself, it is only exercise which is going to shift those pounds. Lemon Balm, mandarin and Lemon should all give you the get up and go needed to get that flab gone! (Use lemon only in a massage oil, putting it in the bath is going to make your eyes water!) By stimulating the body to work with you rather than against you, exercise should really start to pay off.

5. Natural Therapies for Weight Loss

Aromatherapy is the use of concentrated essences of plants to bring about wellness. We call these essences essential oils. They can be extracted from leaves, barks, grasses and flower petals. Each and every one of them has their own special healing abilities.

In this book I cover only the most fundamentals about aromatherapy. If you would like to learn more about the history and the technical side of the art, refer to another of my books *Easy Aromatherapy Recipes For Beginners - An Everyday Guide to Using Simple, Organic and Affordable Essential Oils* which will give you deeper insights into aromatherapy as a whole.

In its truest form aromatherapy is an extremely profound healing skill. A professional aromatherapist is not only an expert in the effects each oil will have but many other aspects of health too. Aromatherapy works on the principle that for a person to feel well, they must be balanced in their mind, their body and their spiritual life too. Essential oils are extremely helpful in bringing about these changes.

As a therapy, it falls under the title of complementary medicine; that is, it is meant to work alongside the traditional medicines which the doctor gives you. It is important never to replace your prescribed medicine with essential oils without consent from your general practitioner. In most cases though, the two treatments work on entirely different body systems and will sit happily together, there are a couple of provisos though.

Essential oils affect blood sugar and the way the body manufactures insulin and so patients with diabetes should avoid some aromatherapy recipes. The same applies for suffers of epilepsy and pregnant women too. This is covered in more detail here.

How to use essential oils

In order to work their magic essential oils need to be absorbed into the body. There are two main ways to do this.

I. Inhalation
II. Through the skin

Inhalation

In some ways the term aromatherapy is a misnomer, as it implies it is the scent of the oils which make them effective. This is not correct. The oils are complex blends of many chemical constituents, each of these create different actions in the body. When we breathe in the oils they travel up the nose via the sinuses, pass through the olfactory system and limbic systems and flush around the brain affecting not only emotions but also releasing hormones too.

The limbic system of our brain is responsible for how we learn, our memories and our emotions. I suppose this is what we would term as our minds.

The sinuses are unusual in that they are the only nerves which travel directly to the brain. All others travel along the spinal cord inside of the spinal column, which means that when oils are inhaled changes in the body will happen very quickly.

This is a wonderful way to affect emotions, to get a quick happy shot or a chill pill, but also it's great for un-bunging stopped up noses too.

Through the Skin

You may see this also described as "trans-dermally", which is the clever kids' version for saying the same thing!

The skin is the largest organ in the body, it also is semi-permeable. The molecules in essential oils are small enough to absorb through the pores of the skin and into the circulatory system. There they flush around the blood stream and go to the parts of the body which need them. These trigger the brain to produce the hormones which balance the body's internal workings and help to bring about healing.

Often when I first started in aromatherapy, twenty years ago, people used to look at me in disbelief and say "so if I rub this cream on my forehead it will cure my headache?" which always seemed a bit odd that they would more readily accept that swallowing a pill might do better. 5 minutes after they had applied the oils you could see their conversion to alternative therapies happening before your very eyes!

In total, it takes around 20 minutes for the skin to fulfil its action of osmosis and for the oils to be fully absorbed.

It is important to remember these oils are *concentrated* essences of plants. They are extremely potent and in some cases will burn the skin. Therefore it is important you always dilute essential oils in some kind of carrier before use.

Discover Carrier oils

The most simplistic of carriers is a standard vegetable oil. There are some beautiful ones on the market all of which have their own wonderfully healing qualities which will enhance essential oils blends. All you need for dilution purposes though is some basic cooking oil, sunflower, grapeseed, or olive perhaps. These make wonderful starting points for massage. The most effective ones you will find for weight loss are Borage and Sea Buckthorn.

Dilution is so small you will wonder whether you have read my notes right, but in 4 fl oz of oil you need no more than 10 drops of essential oils

In The Bath

Putting essential oils in the bath is one of the most effective ways to use them. Remember the skin being an organ, visualize how each pore in the body opens in the warmth of the water and allows the oil access to the body. The warmth softens the muscles and it encourages the capillaries in the skin to move closer to the surface and welcome the oils.

At the same time the steam releases the molecules of the oils into the atmosphere so we can breathe them more easily too, relaxing us and helping us to switch off.

There is only one word we can say really here, isn't there…..aaaaahhhh!

For the full benefit of the aromatherapy bath, lie there for at least 20 minutes.

It is lovely to make bath gifts for birthdays and Christmas but actually there is such a large volume of water in a bath, there is no need for extra carriers. You should use no more than a total of 5 -10 drops into a bath of warm water.

Creams and Lotions

These are very under used, but to my mind they are the single most useful way to carry essential oils. They make great ways to be able to apply small amounts of oils little and often. They protect the skin from the potent oils and they are easy to make and use. You can in effect use any plain cream and stir in some oils, but it is possible to buy blanks from beauty wholesalers and also some pharmacists.

Burners

These are also sometimes called evaporators or diffusers. Some run on electricity, others rely on a candle underneath a bowl of warmed water to release essential oils into the atmosphere. These work really well for changing the atmosphere of a room or for emanating scents which will deter insects, for instance.

DILUTION AND BLENDING

It never ceases to amaze me how many drops of oil people put into a blend. Always employ the philosophy that less is more. This is for two reasons.

   I.   Essential oils are expensive!
   II. The oils are so potent. The body takes what it needs and then releases any surplus into the blood stream as waste. It brings a whole new dimension to throwing money down the toilet!

The very maximum you want to work to is a dilution of 1:25. That is to say for every 25 drops of carrier oil or base you will only want to add 1 drop of essential oil. I work to far less.

Usually one drop of an oil is effective in a blend, two if I want a sledgehammer approach and three drops in emergency situations.

At all times remember you can add more in the next treatment if you need to…but if you get it wrong and add to much you could burn yourself, end up fitting, affect your blood sugar or even your heart. Act sensibly and aromatherapy is your friend, be a fool and I promise you will know about it!!!!

CLAYS

Around the globe there is such a variety of different dirts, dusts and soils we have yet to discover anywhere near all their health benefits. They are extremely detoxifying and cleansing as well as nourishing to the skin. They work directly on the digestive system, so toxins are drawn down into the gut and then eliminated via your stools. For this reason wraps are relaxing and effective and certainly condition the skin but for a faster solution consider purchasing clay in ingestible tablet form. The most effective of these on the market is Betonite Clay

GREEN CLAY

Green Clay is the best choice to make your detoxification wraps. It is extremely cleansing and is effective in purging toxicity out of the body. Use about an ounce (25g) of clay to 1 tsp of carrier oils with essential oil added. Leave a clay wrap on for 20-30 minutes.

RED CLAY or Rhassoul is mined in Morocco and is fabulous for tightening and toning the skin. Use in the same way as is directed for Green Clay.

Clay is a messy business….and then some! It helps to have someone who can apply the clay for you. Covering with clink wrap or a bin bag stops it getting all over the place. I have found the most effective method is to line your empty bath with towels, cover them with a bin bag, lie on the bin bag, put another bag over you, then towels on top. When you are ready to remove the plastic wrap and towels and simply rinse off.

SEA WEED

This has to be the most relaxing and yet most revolting stench of all time, and yet it works fantastically! Sea weed draws toxins out of the system very quickly but also feed your thyroid with iodine too. This a double whammy weight loss gem.

Use three teaspoons of sea weed in a warm bath or use as a wrap as directed with the clays.

SEA SALT THERAPY

This replaces the sea water therapy in Dr Valnet's treatment plan.

Salt is very detoxifying and there are recommendations for both oral uses of salt and for use in the bath.

Sea salt in the bath water improves circulation, rehydrates the skin, improves the skin condition, detoxifies but best of all relaxes!

They also have the added benefit of being amazing at soaking up essential oils. Take 100g of salt (rock salt works well) add 5-10 drops of oil and store in a jar till needed. If you add a drop of food coloring too these make fabulous gifts!

ORAL USE

The secret To 2lb weight loss in just one day.

The disclaimer for oral use is: Ew, ew, ew! It tastes nasty, the effects are nasty, in fact everything about it puts it at the bottom of my desirable-to-do list but since loss of up to 2lb a day is possible, I would be wrong to leave it out.

Recipe: 2tsp Non Iodised Sea Salt

32 Fl oz warm (not hot) water

Add the salt to the water and stir until it is fully dissolved. Try to drink as much as you can in one sitting. It is likely to make you feel very nauseous and windy although flatulence could be a stool, so don't be tempted to give into the urge until you are sitting on the toilet!

The salt very quickly pushes any toxicity through the intestines and you can expect to experience several bouts of diarrhoea as your system rids itself of the accumulated debris. Many people relate experiences of passing what is known as a mucoid plaque, a rope like string of horribleness from the colon, however others suggest that such a thing is, in fact, the stuff of legend. Watch your toilet with interest.

It goes without saying this treatment is not recommended for days when you have to go to work. You need to be able to stay by the lavatory. It is effective from day 1 (which for most people feels like enough cleansing and torture) but can be done safely for up to 3 days.

LYMPHATIC DRAINAGE

Although the lymphatic system is predominately involved in fighting infection it also removes fat from our system as well as fluid. It stands t reason then if we can encourage it to work more effectively we not only immediately lose inches but also speed up the breakdown of fat.

The great news is not only is possible...it is very simple too, using:

LYMPHATIC DRAINAGE MASSAGE

Lymphatic drainage massage the easiest thing in the world. All that is required is to learn to recognise the shift of fluid beneath your fingers and practice how to control it.

Your hands need to maintain a similar position throughout.

Put them side by side and then overlap the thumbs so you have a W shape.

Lay them on the patient and all you need to do is push in the direction of the heart towards the subclavian.

So for puffy ankles:

Start at the ankles and push firmly down pushing up the leg without letting off the pressure. As the fluid starts to accumulate under your hands, take one off and step it back a notch. Let the other one come down and join it but ensure the hands continue to make a dam through which the fluid cannot pass.

Little by little, move the fluid up and when you reach the subclavian gently stroke it over until the build up of fluid has gone. Remember most of the areas of the body empty into the left but there is no hardship if it easier to use the right.

The lymphatic system runs through the entire body so theoretically you can move the lyph anywhere you like. My top tip would always be to start at the ankles and work up, up, up until you have moved all of the fluid you can.

As ever, it seems with this book, stay by the toilet. This time your signal of how well you have moved the fluids will be urination!

ACUPRESSURE POINTS

These are a personal favourite weapon of mine in any type of healing. By using them alongside any other healing mechanism you make it far more potent. In Chinese medicine, acupressure and acupuncture is used to stimulate Qi, the living force energy, to run more freely. Blockages in the flow create dis-ease in the organs. These blockages are painful to the touch and can be "emptied" by applying pressure to the points. Use thumb or a knuckle in circular motions. Be gentle, these points can send patients through the roof; they can be very painful.

Massage any or all of these points for 2/3 minutes at a time.

ABDOMEN: The abdomen point is located three finger breadths below your belly button. Not only will this encourage the body to process your food more effectively, reducing bloating, but it will also ease any constipation.

EAR POINT: This point suppresses appetite. Located close to the ear, open and close your jaw and it is the point which has the most movement.

The fleshy part which connects your earlobe to the rest of the face also contains points which will help to curb appetite.

LIP: Place your thumb inside of your upper lip, (just under the line of your nose) exert pressure with the index finger on the outside of the lip. This is a massage suppressant too.

ELBOW: This is located in the inner crease of your elbow, at the end nearest to you. Stimulating the intestines this helps to remove excess moisture from the body

THE ANKLE: On the inside of each leg, measure two inches up and just off the bone. This is the location of the spleen which kick-starts the digestive system. It suppresses urges to overeat.

Consider integrating these into any of your treatments, massage in particular responds very well here. Be careful not to over stimulate the points. Twice a week for twenty minutes at a time is a good balance.

Phytotherapy and Herbal Suggestions

Milk Thistle
This is the strongest of all the liver cleansing herbals.

Chorella
This algae helps the body to expel heavy metal poisons. A recent Japanese study demonstrated its amazing weight loss qualities were attributed to chorella's ability to speed up metabolism. Because it is nutritionally such a complete meal, you feel very full after taking it.

Kelp
The jury is still out as to whether kelp helps everyone lose weight. Its impressive iodine content means it will make definite improvements to poor metabolic activity due to thyroid dysfunction. That aside, most practitioners agree the added benefits of thicker hair and stronger nails make it a gamble worth taking.

Anti Cellulite Diet
For some women even months and months of strict dieting and gruelling gym hours will not succeed in improving the unsightly orange peel skin which we call know as cellulite. I have seem a treatment blend of essential oils combined with lymphatic drainage and 28 days with the following dietary restrictions have extremely impressive results; the treatment plan succeeds where all else fails.

Remove all red meat, cheese and dairy, alcohol, sugar, tea and coffee.

Increase water intake to help with rehydration and elimination of toxicity.

6. HOUSEKEEPING

Buying Essential Oils

It seems proper at this point to explain my comment earlier that essential oils are expensive. It is true, but there are good reasons for it. There are many factors which affect their prices.

These are:

I. Method of extraction – CO_2 costs far more than expression
II. Yield – some plants only generate small amounts of oil so far more plant matter is required.
III. Availability of plant matter – Some plants are seasonal or only grow in certain places
IV. Sustainable resources- Oils such as sandalwood have to be gained from specially grown trees.
V. Dilution – Some oils are what are called "cut" with other oils to make them easier for people to afford to buy. A good example of this is Lemon Balm oil or Melissa officianalis. Melissa (True) is 100% pure, Melissa (Type) has been cut with Lemon Verbena oil because Lemon balm leaves are notoriously hard to get much oil from.

All of these dictate how much an oil will cost you. Essential oil production is a huge economy but actually oil retailing prices do not vary that much, it is not particularly competitive. It is fair to say if a price seems lower than any others you have seen…there is probably a reason to think it may be of inferior quality.

Labelling should give you some pointers. Always check that the oil is shown with its English name but also its Latin name too. You should see it shown as *Lavendula latifolia.* Note how the first word is shown with a capital letter and the second is in small case? If a label differs from this there may be cause for concern. This method of labelling (called binomial nomenclature) will tell you which species of the family of plants an oil has been taken from.

In some parts of the world and especially on some MLM marketing websites, you may also see essential oils graded. You may see them denoted as *Grade A* or *therapeutic grade* oils. This is purely a marketing ploy; no such official legislation has ever been introduced.

The French, who are some of the planet's most prolific oil producers, have some governance from an organisation called AFNOR. This can be used as a guide to show you quality of the oil but not necessarily for therapeutic reasons. Afnor is solely concerned with the quality of the oil for the economic growth of the areas for export.

Your label will often show country of origin and this can be useful. Some areas of production naturally have less pollution and so are more pure. An Alpine lavender plant will be grown at such altitude it is way above the rigours of pollution. There are fewer of these plants and so this comes at a high price tag.

By contrast think of the scary things which pour into the soil and the air in war zones...oils taken from these areas tend to have sharpness to them from the pollution they have absorbed.

Look for organic oils for this reason; they are purer and more effective. As discussed before, if a label says CO2 extracted you have found a rather beautiful thing. You should give your purse a good shake and see if you can find a few extra pennies to spend on it.

STORING ESSENTIAL OILS

When we start all of us make the same mistake. In fact, remember I have said this as you clear up your first mess! Essential oils degrade plastic. If you store a blend in a plastic bottle, sooner or later it is going to melt into a revolting greasy mess in your cupboard!

Store all essential oils products in dark glass bottles in a dark place.

Just like all organisms, plant essences are subject to oxidation. Over time the cells begin to die off and the oils lose their efficacy. Some oils oxidise faster than others. Citrus oils for instance begin to degrade after just 6 months. On the other hand I have a bottle of myrrh oil which is still going strong 15 years after I got it....it works but it's not got superman strength any longer.

Sunlight is like kryptonite to oils. It oxidises them far faster than anything else. Keep them dark and keep them cool.

When you do undo the top to use the oils, be aware that they are volatile and so molecules are escaping even if you are not pouring drops. Ensure you put the lid back on tight enough to stop the escape further.

Ensure you wash your hands after use (think about forgetting to wash chilli off your fingers and then rubbing your eyes but ten times as bad!) In fact, I think my experience of rushing to the loo with citronella oil on my hands may have been even worse than that! Lordie....my eyes did run!!!!

Lastly, keep essential oils out of reach of children. Every one of my kids has loved having "Magic Eels" in the bath, and then thought about adding some themselves when I've not been looking. The wrong oil in the bath can do just as much damage as scalding water. Worse too, some oils smell like sweeties. Remember Parma Violets? Violet oil smells exactly the same. Leaving essential oils around when there are curious fingers is a recipe for disaster.

Safety Advice

Essential oils are not suitable for everyone. The way they encourage the hormones in the systems to alter can create damaging effects in some groups.

The main people to have concerns are:

Diabetes

People with diabetes can safely use most essential oils with the exception of angelica oil. Oils which encourage the pancreas to work more effectively are dill and fennel and as such these are very helpful to suffers.

Epilepsy

Some essential oils are what is called neuro-toxic which makes them dangerous not only to suffers of epilepsy but also some types of schizophrenia too. Essential oils to avoid are: Rosemary, fennel, sage, eucalyptus, hyssop, camphor and spike lavender (Lavendula latifolia)

Pregnant Women

Using essential oils for weight loss when you are pregnant is not advised as many of the oils can affect fluid loss which is vital to the baby.

Breast Feeding

Whilst essential oils are safe whilst breast feeding, they do affect the taste of the milk. Some babies simply don't enjoy them. If baby does go off the milk, leave oils off for a day to see if she takes up the milk again.

7. Recipes

Aromatherapy is by no means an exact science and this book equips you with plenty of knowledge and expertise to create your own recipes based on the challenges you face at any given time on your diet. What follows are just few simple ideas to help you see how the different ways the oils can be used. Get excited and get experimenting.

WILLPOWER EVAPORATOR OIL
1 drop Mandarin

1 drop Lavender

1 drop Citronella

Use in a burner to affect your mood.

RESILIENCE LOTION
100 ml Blank Lotion

2 drops Sweet Fennel

2 drops Helichrism

1 drop Rose Maroc

Mix together and apply a finger full three times a day to either the insides of the wrists, or any of the acupressure points which help reduce hunger cravings.

ENVIRONMENTAL CLEANSING MASSAGE OIL
100 ml Grapeseed Oil

2 Drops Sweet Fennel

2 drops Tagetes

1 drop Ginger

1 drop Basil

1 drop Sandalwood

Use twice a day before meals, gently massaging the oil directly onto the abdomen. Stroke into the skin, circling the belly button in a clockwise direction, to mimic the digestive journey.

FAT BURNING LOTION
3 drops Grapefruit

1 drop Sweet Fennel

1 drop Ginger

Use 20 minutes before eating on the inside of the wrists.

Bye Bye Hunger Pangs Lotion (For Daytime Use)
100 ml blank lotion

2 drops peppermint

2 drops ginger

1 drop frankincense

Use as and when required either on the wrists, rubbed into the back of the neck for speedy access to the brain, or over appropriate acupressure points. Experiment to see which method best suits you as an individual.

Bye Bye Hunger Pangs Lotion (For Evening Use)
100 ml blank lotion

2 drops lavender

1 drop camomile roman

2 drops ginger

1 drop frankincense

Use as above. This recipe has peppermint omitted as it will keep you awake at night.

STRESS CLEANSE
This blend is designed to fortify the liver and adrenals after long term stress and then nourish it to kick start the fat burning processes.

100 ml blank lotion

2 x Mandarin

2 x Camomile Maroc

1 x Peppermint

2 x Eucalyptus

1 x Rosemary (omit if there are issues with epilepsy)

3 x Cardomom

Use a small finger full three times a day, on the inside of the wrists.

INCH LOSS WRAP
25 g Green Clay

1 tsp Borage Carrier Oil

2 drops Sweet Fennel

3 drops Cypress

3 drops Grapefruit

2 drops Juniper

I recommend taking before and after measurements with this one. It will definitely make you smile!

Apply over the area which requires shrinkage! Cover with cling film to avoid too much mess. Leave on for 30 minutes.

Rinse away thoroughly. Follow with skin tightening gel.

SKIN TIGHTENING GEL
100 mls Glycolic Gel (available from beauty wholesalers)

1 drop Black Pepper

3 drops Geranium

2 drops Cypress

2 drops Juniper

1 drop Helichrysm

Smear over the skin like a masque. It should rub in quite well, but it works better to smear on "too much" and let it soak in for around 20 minutes.

Conclusion

Hopefully by the time you reach this page you have been elated by the tape measure and scales already. I wish you well in your smaller jeans!

Before I go though, I would like to ask you consider how miraculous a medicine you have discovered. Plants evolve and develop to match the needs of the planet. How amazing we should have some of these incredible gifts in our back yards.

As you feel stronger and fitter, why not take up a spade or a fork and dig over a small patch of your own garden for some herbs. There never was a better exercise and in turn will do your own part in healing our world. Provide a little oxygen for our children's children, so they too can experience the healing joys of the plants of their own time.

BIBLIOGRAPHY

The author would like to thank the writers of the following text books and websites for the insights they have given to this research.

Robert Tisserand – The Art of Aromatherapy

Patricia Davis – Aromatherapy an A-Z

Jill Bruce – The Garden of Eden

Elizabeth Ashley – How To Overcome Diabetes Naturally

Michael Cook – Environmental Toxins and Medical Dowsing

Dr Jean Valnet – The Practice of Aromatherapy

Valerie Ann Worwood – Aromantics

Natalie Kent – The Mind Body Connections

Thanks for reading!

I do hope you enjoyed this book. If you did, you could help support me most of all with an honest review on Amazon!

Just visit Amazon.com and click: Order History

DISCLAIMER
by SEQ Legal

---

(1) Introduction

This disclaimer governs the use of this ebook. [By using this ebook, you accept this disclaimer in full. / We will ask you to agree to this disclaimer before you can access the ebook.]

(2) Credit

This disclaimer was created using an SEQ Legal template.

(3) No advice

The ebook contains information about aromatherapy and the use of essential oils. The information is not advice, and should not be treated as such.

[You must not rely on the information in the ebook as an alternative to qualified medical advice from a health professional. advice from an appropriately qualified professional. If you have any specific questions about any medical matter you should consult an appropriately qualified professional.]

[If you think you may be suffering from any medical condition you should seek immediate medical attention. You should never delay seeking medical advice, disregard medical advice, or discontinue medical treatment because of information in the ebook.]

(4)   No representations or warranties

To the maximum extent permitted by applicable law and subject to section 6 below, we exclude all representations, warranties, undertakings and guarantees relating to the ebook.

Without prejudice to the generality of the foregoing paragraph, we do not represent, warrant, undertake or guarantee:

> that the information in the ebook is correct, accurate, complete or non-misleading;

> that the use of the guidance in the ebook will lead to any particular outcome or result; or

> in particular, that by using the guidance in the ebook you will heal disease or work in any way as a cure for illness.

(5) Limitations and exclusions of liability

The limitations and exclusions of liability set out in this section and elsewhere in this disclaimer: are subject to section 6 below; and govern all liabilities arising under the disclaimer or in relation to the ebook, including liabilities arising in contract, in tort (including negligence) and for breach of statutory duty.

We will not be liable to you in respect of any losses arising out of any event or events beyond our reasonable control.

We will not be liable to you in respect of any business losses, including without limitation loss of or damage to profits, income, revenue, use, production, anticipated savings, business, contracts, commercial opportunities or goodwill.

We will not be liable to you in respect of any loss or corruption of any data, database or software.

We will not be liable to you in respect of any special, indirect or consequential loss or damage.

(6) Exceptions

Nothing in this disclaimer shall: limit or exclude our liability for death or personal injury resulting from negligence; limit or exclude our liability for fraud or fraudulent misrepresentation; limit any of our liabilities in any way that is not permitted under applicable law;

or exclude any of our liabilities that may not be excluded under applicable law.

(7) Severability

If a section of this disclaimer is determined by any court or other competent authority to be unlawful and/or unenforceable, the other sections of this disclaimer continue in effect.

If any unlawful and/or unenforceable section would be lawful or enforceable if part of it were deleted, that part will be deemed to be deleted, and the rest of the section will continue in effect.

(8) Law and jurisdiction

This disclaimer will be governed by and construed in accordance with English law, and any disputes relating to this disclaimer will be subject to the exclusive jurisdiction of the courts of England and Wales.

Made in the USA
Lexington, KY
18 April 2015